A Practical Guide to Addison's & Adrenal Fatigue

Advice for dealing with Addison's/adrenal fatigue from a female over-achiever diagnosed at 31.

This is the result of recognizing a need for a practical life guide for Addison's/adrenal fatigue patients. Addison's is considered rare; the frequency rate estimated at either one in 100,000 or 40-60 cases per million and all the estimates are considered problematic at best.

Disclaimer: I make some bold statements about what you should do. That's because of a mix of my personality and being convinced this approach has worked for me. I'm not a doctor, but I do think I'm smart enough to be one.

Regan J. Heineke

It should be understood that it is written for anyone with adrenals performing in a less than optimal manner in the hopes you might reverse any progression you have towards full-blown failure.

"Addison's disease" is historically the term for complete adrenal failure that requires life-long replacement of adrenal function. I, however, have first-hand experience that it is not all or nothing and believe this strict definition is the result of insurance companies looking for any reason not to cover patients. I fit the profile for a primary Addison's diagnosis (my basal cortisol level was <20 mcg/dL and increased 7.1 mcg/dL after doing the ACTH stimulation test); however, I tested negative to the adrenal antibody (and have also tested negative for all physical reasons for secondary Addison's). I have proven adrenal insufficiency that causes me to have the exact same symptoms and outcomes as someone with this strictly defined diagnosis, but I do not fit the classic Addison's profile that would allow me to access the full range of insurance coverage.

For this reason, I do not discriminate between "Addison's disease" and "adrenal fatigue/failure" and use both terms throughout this document.

Regan J. Heineke

Table of Contents

Take Home Message: Be Kind to Your Adrenal Glands

Your adrenal glands do not produce sufficient hormones (baseline and in response to physical or emotional stress), meaning you have to compromise what you use your finite amount of cortisol for each day and your ability to recover is compromised. You must avoid anything that stimulates your adrenal glands/sends them the signal that they should work and need to build in extra recovery time and energy for every little thing. Even seemingly minimal mental stress will have you fatigued, aggravated, sweaty, and/or nauseous.

About Adrenal Glands

Adrenal glands release hormones in response to stress (the subjective feeling of pressure and/or the many objective physiological responses to physical and emotional stressors) by synthesizing cholesterol. The following are produced in the adrenal cortex:

1. Aldosterone in the outermost layer – zona glomerulosa
2. Cortisol in the middle layer – zona fasciculate
3. DHEA, progesterone, and androstenedione in the inner most layer – zona reticularis

The adrenal medulla – the core of the adrenal gland surrounded by the adrenal cortex – secretes noradrenaline and adrenaline.

Synthesis Pathway
(all hormones synthesized from cholesterol):

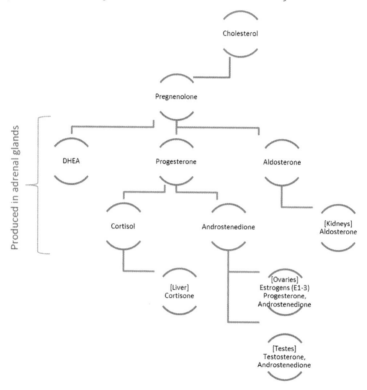

[ ] Indicates organ hormones are used by.

The Descent into Addison's/Adrenal Fatigue

Whether you have primary (autoimmune) or secondary (some other physical cause) Addison's, chances are you have been experiencing the symptoms of adrenal fatigue for some time. You've probably noticed something's off but have attributed your symptoms to other, more common causes (i.e. not eating as well as you should, a lingering cold, drank a little too much, exercised a little too much, etc.). Symptoms are often nonspecific (i.e. fatigue, weakness, nausea, abdominal pain, gastroenteritis, mood variations), which makes a diagnosis difficult. The book "Adrenal Fatigue: The 21st Century Stress Syndrome" by James L. Wilson, N.D., D.C., Ph.D. contains a Health History Timeline that is helpful for revealing how all your issues and symptoms are attributable to your adrenal glands.

Stage 1

Your body mounts an aggressive anti-stress response to stress including an increase in producing and releasing cortisol. Your symptoms are mild and can be "fixed" by more coffee, sugar, and/or carbohydrates.

Stage 2

The adrenals are unable to keep up with the cortisol demand. Your fatigue is pronounced at night and despite a full night's rest, you do not feel refreshed. Anxiety and irritability are noticeable. You are catching more colds than normal, and if you are female, your menstrual cycle is irregular either in timing or experience. You have probably started to tell your doctor about your symptoms.

Stage 3

The adrenals cannot keep up with the demand for cortisol and become exhausted. Baseline cortisol output declines. You are chronically fatigued, have foggy thoughts, struggle to exercise, have adrenaline rushes, erratic blood pressure, anxiety attacks, low libido, and slow digestion. You are able to relatively recover after a day or two of rest.

Stage 4:

Your body has realized there is not enough cortisol and you are in shock. You are having severe cardiovascular issues, lower back pain, vomiting and/or diarrhea, dehydration, and loss of consciousness.

Addisonian Crisis

An Addisonian crisis (a.k.a. adrenal crisis, acute adrenal insufficiency) is a life-threatening state caused by insufficient levels of cortisol, which are necessary to regulate blood sugar, suppress the immune response, and react to stress. Hospitalization, corticosteroids and intravenous fluids to support low blood pressure, and monitoring is required. Symptoms of a crisis include:

- Headache
- Fatigue/ profound weakness
- Slow, sluggish movement
- Nausea/ vomiting
- Low blood pressure
- Dehydration
- High fever
- Shaking chills
- Confusion or coma
- Darkening of the skin
- Rapid heart rate
- Joint pain

- Abdominal pain
- Unintentional weight loss
- Rapid respiratory rate
- Unusual/ excessive sweating on face and/or palms

- Loss of appetite
- Elevated potassium in blood
- Low sodium in blood

My Story

Early Warning Signs I Missed:

3-4 years prior...	My upper lip area darkened unexpectedly, looking as though I had a tan in just this spot, but it was not summer. Face creams did not alleviate it.
2 years prior...	I periodically experienced night sweats and insomnia, which I attributed to a recent breakup.
18 months prior...	I had an unusual and severe hangover that was not explained by the amount of alcohol I had consumed. It took three days to fully recover and from then on I had decreased alcohol tolerance.
1 year prior...	I noticed an increase in my salt cravings. Prior to this point I had been slowly cutting manufactured sodium out of my diet and was never a salt lover. After this point my salt craving was insatiable.
3 months prior...	I ended up in the hospital with severe food poisoning, which did not make any sense because my brother ate the same meal but did not have any reaction. It took five days to recover, even after an IV and medication in the hospital.
1 month prior...	I developed very noticeable dark spots and a dark line near the hairline on my forehead.

You with Addison's/Adrenal Fatigue

As mentioned, I am convinced that adrenal fatigue and Addison's are one in the same even though the pharmaceutical/insurance complex does not recognize them as similar. The outcome of adrenal fatigue is the same as Addison's: your adrenal glands do not produce sufficient hormones (baseline and in response to physical or emotional stress). The only difference is that if you have the primary (autoimmune) version or even certain secondary versions, your adrenals will never recover.

Regardless of how you came to have Addison's/adrenal fatigue, here is what you can expect with it:

- *Fatigue/crashing without recovering.*
  When you get tired you cannot re-energize and may have a headache that no amount of water or aspirin relieves. For the most part naps do not remedy the fatigue. Your body is struggling to cope and it seems endless.

- *Poor sleeping.*
  Both high and low nighttime cortisol levels can interrupt sound sleep. Circulating cortisol normally rises (typically highest ~8am) and falls throughout the day (lowest between midnight and 4am). You do not get the benefit of high morning cortisol and you probably used what little cortisol you did have throughout the day, meaning you probably have abnormally low cortisol at night.

- *Unexplained fear/anxiety.*
  Low cortisol levels cause anxiety, irritability, an inability to handle stress, fatigue, and feeling overwhelmed. In addition, depression has been associated with both elevated and low levels of cortisol.

- *Chronically low blood pressure and trouble regulating blood pressure changes.*
  This is because your lack of cortisol means you cannot appropriately regulate sodium and potassium. This is also why you're so thirsty and your heart sometimes races.

- *Caffeine sensitivity.*
  Caffeine tells your adrenal glands to release cortisol, which you are no longer capable of, and so you start heading towards a crisis.

- *Hypoglycemia/an uncomfortable reaction to sugars/carbohydrates.*
  Cortisol plays an important role in maintaining blood sugar levels. The adrenals fail to raise blood sugar (glucose) levels enough to meet the increased demand. The lack of cortisol also reduces insulin resistance in your cells, depleting your available energy further.

> **My Story**
>
> Anxiety disorders run in my family so I accepted my constant background anxiousness as a fact of my life.
>
> As soon as I started taking cortisol I felt an overwhelming sense of contentment that I cannot remember having as an adult. I can finally "turn off" my worrying. I'm confident life will work out in my favor.

- *Food sensitivities/allergies.*
  Under-performing adrenal glands make you more susceptible to sensitivities/allergies that you never had, or increase your reactions to allergies you already had.

- *Anger/irritability.*
  Your adrenal glands produce and regulate adrenaline and noradrenaline – your fight or flight response. Stress that you considered minimal before can now quickly put you in a rage.

- *Decreased mental capacity.*
  The cortisol and aldosterone imbalances result in abnormal blood pressure, which starves your brain of the nutrients it needs to function normally.

- *Increased negative reaction to heat.*
  Heat dehydrates you and increases your fatigue, and then you have a hard time recovering.

- *Easy bruising.*
  A very visible outcome of your inability to recover normally is easy bruising that is darker and lasts longer than normal.

- *Skin darkening.*
  Excess ACTH binds to dermal melanocytes, which change the color of pigment to a dark brown or black. Hyperpigmentation usually occurs on sun-exposed areas of the skin, knuckles, elbows, knees, and scars formed after Addison's. The vaginal and perianal mucosa may be affected.

Tests You'll Want
Adrenal insufficiency can manifest as a defect anywhere in the hypothalamic-pituitary-adrenal axis so you'll want to keep testing along this axis until you find an answer.

- Antibody tests to see if you are having an autoimmune response:
    - Adrenal, pituitary, and thyroid
        - Note: the antibody tests are not 100% accurate. You can test negative and still actually have the autoimmune version.

- ACTH Stimulation Test:
    - This is the most specific test for diagnosing adrenal insufficiency. Blood cortisol levels are measured before and after a synthetic form of ACTH is injected. This test quantifies your adrenal insufficiency and can distinguish whether the cause is adrenal (low cortisol/aldosterone production) or pituitary (low ACTH production).

- Hormone curves/baseline tests.
  Note: hormone ranges are an art, not a science. Unless you have had previous hormone curve/baseline tests, you will struggle to interpret what the results mean for you. However, these tests contribute to the overall picture of your hormone situation and you will have future curves/baselines to compare them to.

- Insulin-Induced Hypoglycemia Test:
    - This test is used to determine how the hypothalamus, pituitary, and adrenal glands respond to stress. Blood is drawn to measure the blood glucose and cortisol levels, followed by an injection of fast-acting insulin. Blood glucose and cortisol levels are measured again 30, 45, and 90 minutes after the insulin injection. The normal response is for blood glucose levels to fall (this represents the stress) and cortisol levels to rise.

- Tumor Markers:
    - If there is a cancerous tumor, tumor markers will be found in your blood or urine.

- Imaging (CT, MRI, Ultrasound) to see if any part of your glands have been physically degraded:
    - Adrenal, pituitary, and thyroid

- Blood Culture:
    - If you are fighting an infection, bacteria will be found in your blood.

- Other tests to ensure you're not stressing your body:
    - Food sensitivity/allergy
    - Celiac's
    - Vitamin deficiencies – especially B12. Vitamin B deficiencies are common with adrenal gland issues. In fact, a blood disorder caused by a lack of vitamin B12 used to be known as "Addison's anemia."

My Story

I tested sensitive to 19 foods, 13 of which I ate regularly. I was skeptical of their impact, but I have noticed an improvement with my new diet.

Mild racing heart was common after my preferred breakfast (consisting almost entirely of foods I'm sensitive to), which I attributed to low morning cortisol levels. With my new diet, I rarely experience morning racing heart and am able to regularly skip my second dose of hydrocortisone.

After eliminating all sensitive foods for three months I am able to occasionally eat the foods I am sensitive to without experiencing racing heart or fatigue.

If your adrenal glands are not functioning or not functioning properly, treatment will consist of lifestyle changes (to reduce the demand on your adrenals), pharmaceutical treatments (to stabilize your hormone activity), and naturopathic treatments (to encourage your body's own healing processes).

Lifestyle Changes You Need to Make

I have been able to remain stable on an impressively low dose of steroid hormones and I believe that is due to my significant lifestyle changes. The goal is to live your life in a way that requires minimal effort from your adrenal glands. If you're like me, this way of life is significantly different from than the life you lived before you realized you had adrenal gland issues.

Eliminate Indefinitely

Waking Up to an Alarm
Just like with caffeine, you do not want to send unnatural signals to your adrenal glands by waking up before your body sends the signal that it is time to wake up. To understand this concept, it is important to understand the daily cortisol curve. In general, cortisol peaks at 8am, dips at 11 am – 12 pm and again at 2-4 pm, and starts to fall at 8 pm until it nearly zeroes out from midnight – 4 am.

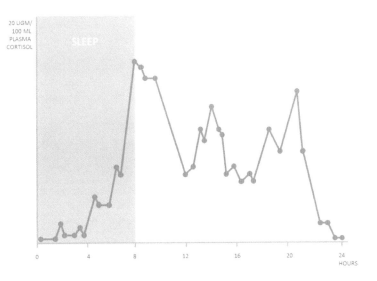

When you set an alarm before ~8 am and force yourself out of bed, your adrenals get the signal to increase cortisol production. Even if you are taking replacement cortisol, you have a very limited amount of cortisol to use each day and should spend it on more important life stressors than waking up before you are ready.

Staying up past 10 pm

Just like caffeine and not waking up to an alarm, you do not want to send unnatural signals to your adrenal glands that they need to produce extra cortisol because you are still awake after ~10 pm. The peak of cortisol ~8 pm and then its steep decline until ~10 pm sends a consistent signal to your body that it is time to sleep. Ignoring this signal deprives you of the most beneficial hours of sleep – between 10 pm and 2 am.

Even if you are not asleep, you should be in bed and resting as though you were sleeping by 10 pm each night. This consistent behavior will train all of your body's processes to fall in line with your daily hormone cycle. Avoid large meals in the evening as the digestion activities – and associated release of hormones – make sleep more difficult.

My Story
During my stabilization period, I was typically ready for bed ~9pm, but would wake up again ~11pm (sometimes with night sweats), and struggle with light sleep and nightmares throughout the night.

After my diagnosis, I realized that for the prior year I was having a chronically high cortisol sleeping problem – my body and mind was just wired at night and I could not genuinely rest.

Caffeine

Caffeine stimulates the adrenal glands to increase cortisol release. At its core, this is an unnatural signal to your adrenal glands and causes them to work "overtime." Even if you are taking replacement cortisol, you have a very limited amount of cortisol to use each day and should spend it on more important life stressors. Finally, caffeine causes dehydration, which exacerbates the hypoadrenocorticism from Addison's (the inability to balance salt and potassium and therefore blood pressure and fluid balance). Caffeine comes in many forms:

- Coffee (even 8 oz. of decaf has 2-12 mg)

- Cocoa

- "Energy" drinks, bars, supplements, and miscellaneous food products

- Soda

- Black, green, and iced tea

- Some medications such as Excedrin

Sugar

Fake sugar or high amounts of carbohydrates (candy, cookies, sodas, processed foods, white bread, etc.) causes an inflammatory response in your body, which tells your adrenal glands to release more cortisol as cortisol prevents the release of substances in the body that cause inflammation. Of all the things you will need to spend your limited amount of cortisol on (i.e. the cold going around), this one is completely unnecessary. If your recipe calls for sugar, substitute with honey or molasses in small amounts. Avoid the following fake sugars:

- Dextrose
- Dextrin
- Lactose
- Maltose
- Sucrose
- Fructose

- Modified food starch
- Corn syrup
- Corn sweetener
- Cornstarch

- Natural sweetener
- Sorbitol
- Hexanol
- Mannitol
- Glycol

Hunger

Cortisol controls blood sugar levels and is essential to maintaining normal body function (metabolism). Cortisol also affects several hormones responsible for hunger and cravings (leptin, insulin, and neuropeptide). Hunger is stressful for your body, which tells your adrenal glands to release more cortisol. It is important to eat regularly throughout the day to avoid any feelings of hunger that will stress your body. Establishing a regular meal schedule that your body can rely on stabilizes blood sugar, which stabilizes all the processes reliant on proper blood sugar levels. Even within your schedule, you should always eat as needed. It is particularly important to eat soon after waking because it is when your lack of cortisol production is most pronounced and your body is in most need of nourishment.

Eliminate Somewhat Indefinitely

Heavy/Intense Aerobic Activities

It is important to note that exercise is very healthy for the Addison's patient and should be continued. However, intense exercise causes physical stress, which tells your adrenal glands to release more cortisol. Remember that your cortisol demand continues after you're done exercising – you need further cortisol to repair and replenish. Additionally, exercise can cause dehydration, which exacerbates your inability to balance salt and potassium and therefore blood pressure and fluid balance.

Cut out heavy exercise at first and replace it with gentle activities such as yoga and walking. As you feel better, gradually increase the intensity and duration of the exercising. Do not schedule back-to-back heavy exercises as you need extra time to recover. Be extremely responsive to your body's needs. If you feel even slightly awkward, stop. Finally, stay positive about every exercise attempt. Even if you were not able to do all you had hoped to do, you are taking a positive step towards reaching your exercise goals.

My Story
During my stabilization period I occasionally tried to attend my high-intensity, high-interval training class. I would make it through the class alright, but I would crash afterwards...to the point of having blurry vision.

After stabilization and learning to time my steroid cortisol dose so that I'm flush with cortisol before exercising, I am able to attend the high-intensity class once a week as long as I am enjoying good health from all of my other lifestyle changes.

Alcohol

While some studies have reported that low doses of alcohol may reduce the response to a stressor, other studies have shown alcohol may stimulate hormone release by the hypothalamus, pituitary, and adrenal glands. While alcohol's effect in your body is highly dependent on multiple genetic and environmental factors and you should carefully weigh the pros and cons, we do know that alcohol causes dehydration, which exacerbates your inability to balance salt and potassium and therefore blood pressure and fluid balance.

If you have consumed enough alcohol to cause a hangover, your body will require additional cortisol for recovery. For each alcoholic drink you consume, follow it with a glass of water or sports drink to replace the fluids you will lose. This means that you will not experience drunkenness, which is essentially dehydration. If you are also dealing with hyper/hypoglycemia, alcohol interferes with all three sources of glucose and the hormones needed to maintain healthy blood glucose levels.

As with the above items, there are better things to spend your limited amount of cortisol on.

Adrenaline-Inducing Activities

Positive events also can be stressful. Roller coasters, haunted houses, action and horror films, competition, etc., etc., require your adrenal glands to react to stress. Avoid these activities until you feel stable enough to introduce them back into your life in small doses.

Reduce

Stress

Psychological or emotional stress from any source can cause an Addisonian crisis with the same effectiveness as physical stress or illness. Most endocrinologists recommend the same increase in steroid dose during psychological stress and emotional upsets as they do during physical stress or physical illness. Your brain perceives stress as a threat and signals your body to release a burst of hormones.

It is important that you reduce both personal and professional sources of stress. You have a finite amount of cortisol to spend each day (that is never enough) to handle stress. You will need to severely reduce the list of stressors you are willing to compromise your health on. You will then need to prioritize the remaining stressors and strictly limit yourself to only dealing with one stress at a time.

Once you start monitoring your stress, you will learn to recognize and avoid your stress triggers. Identify which aspect of the situation you can control as a starting point. Remember that stress interferes with your productivity and impact. Treating your body and mind with patience and compassion can only improve your work product.

Do not fall into the trap of feeling like you have to figure it out all on your own. Seek help and support from family and friends.

My Story

My career is a constant flow of 1-2 week deadlines, my team is very lean, and we handle a comparatively large workload.

I was very concerned about what I perceived to be a physical limitation on my work productivity. However, my actual experience has been the exact opposite. I am handling the same volume of work and my diagnosis has forced me to ensure that every step I take is as efficient as possible. Due to my focus on living a relaxed lifestyle, I approach each project with a clearer, more focused, and positive mindset. Coworkers have even commented that I have become more open-minded and approachable.

Add

Sports Drinks

To combat your low blood pressure and do all you can to assist your body in its attempts to balance salt and potassium, regularly drink a sugar-free sports drink that either has sodium or that you've added salt to. I recommend Vitamin Water Zero in orange flavor (as it has an acceptable sugar type/amount and potassium) with Himalayan pink salt added. Himalayan pink salt is the "healthiest salt" available as it contains the same 84 trace minerals and elements, has less sodium per serving, and exists in a form small enough for cells to easily absorb. If you are on steroid hormones and experiencing minor infections (i.e. dermatitis, yeast infections, etc.) also add a tablespoon of apple cider vinegar.

Water

Addison's disease affects the balance of water, sodium, and potassium in the body. To help combat this reality, increase your water intake. However, you also want to avoid over-hydrating. When you drink too much water, the level of sodium in the blood falls and causes dehydration. Watch for these signs of dehydration and respond quickly:

- Dry mouth/thirst
- Sleepy/tired
- Decreased urine output
- Few/no tears
- Dry skin
- Headache
- Constipation
- Dizzy/lightheaded

Healthy Eating

When dealing with any ailment you want to ensure your body has the nutrition it needs to perform. Proper nutrition is doubly important with adrenal dysfunction because nutritional deficiencies cause physical stress. Part of healthy eating is also eating regularly and having positive food experiences. Consider taking a probiotic to increase your ability to absorb nutrients in the proper amounts.

What to Eat

Whole Foods

Increase your vegetable intake and reduce the consumption of empty calories. Look for foods with low sugar and fat content that have complex carbohydrates and eat with a balanced amount of protein[1]. Whole grains, fruits, vegetables, nuts, and seeds are high in vitamins and minerals need for your immune system. Eat fruit in moderation as it can be high in sugar even though the fiber helps the body absorb the sugar more slowly. Remember that you are doing your best to eliminate sugar, including carbohydrates. Most carbohydrates turn into blood sugar, with liquid carbohydrates being absorbed quicker than solid carbohydrates.

---

[1] However, if you are on steroid medications you may need to increase protein intake as steroids affect the metabolism of calcium and vitamin D and can lead to bone loss. It is important to note the rates of bone loss differ depending on the individual and the size of the dose.

Organic

Organic foods are preferable as it gives you a better chance of avoiding synthetic chemicals and food additives that may unnaturally influence your hormone levels. Of the estimated 3,000 additives used in the United States to preserve foods or improve their taste and appearance, only about 2,000 have detailed toxicological information available. Also avoid unnatural food packaging. For example, synthetic xenoestrogens are widely used in plastic bottles and can linings. The Endocrine Society regards them as serious environmental hazards that have hormone disruptive effects on both wildlife and humans.

Anti-Inflammatory

As mentioned in the "Tests You'll Want" section, avoid eating foods you are allergic or sensitive to and rotate/add variety often. Allergic reactions not only require your adrenals to respond to a stressful event, they also damage the intestines and reduce absorption of the food's nutrients. Unfortunately poorly functioning adrenal glands increase your risk of allergies. Cortisol controls the level of inflammatory reactions in the body. You will likely find that you have developed new allergies/sensitivities.

How to Eat

Frequently
Unfortunately adrenal fatigue (and taking steroid hormones) leads to blood sugar imbalances (hyperglycemia or hypoglycemia depending on your cortisol levels). Never skip a meal and eat a high-fiber, low-sugar snack whenever you are the least bit hungry. Snack more frequently during times of increased mental, emotional, or physical stress.

Diversely
Constantly change the type of food you are eating. The less you eat of one particular food, the less likely you are to become allergic to it since most food allergies are dose-related (turn on the food- antibody response). Eating a variety of food also increases your chances of ingesting the variety of nutrients your body needs to heal.

Patiently
Finally, treat your meals as relaxation time. Chew your food well and eat slowly. This signals your body to slow the digestive response (less stress) and allows you to absorb more nutrients from your food.

Relaxation Techniques
Your adrenal glands will benefit from daily practice of stress-reduction techniques such as deep breathing, massage, yoga, practicing mindfulness, meditation, and/or being in nature.

Naps

Do not fight your fatigue. Your body is telling you that it requires rest for recovery. Listen to your body and respond by resting. You have every reason to be tired and your body will reward you by repairing and recovering.

Emotional Responsiveness

Just like responding to your physical need for rest and recovery, you must respond positively to your emotional needs. This is doubly difficult for the Addison's patient because they already have increased levels of anxiety, fear, and over-reactions to stimuli, and may have a history of putting their emotional needs last. As mentioned, psychological or emotional stress can cause an Addisonian crisis and require an increase in steroid dose. Especially while you are in recovery, it is important to recognize and resolve emotional stress. Do whatever you need to do to remain content and positive.

Pharmaceutical Treatments

Treatment includes replacing the hormones you no longer make with synthetic steroid hormones. The treatment of Addison's often focuses on cortisol as its effects are far-reaching and systemic and play many roles in maintaining homeostasis. As a result of your body's inability to control cortisol, you will also need to take a steroid that balances fluid and electrolytes. However, low cortisol may not be your only hormone issue and you will want to encourage your doctor to treat your entire hormone situation. The correct dose (type and amount) of replacement hormones is far more of an art than a science.

The goal of your treatment is to allow your adrenal glands to rest and recover. You do not want to over- or under-suppress them. All synthetic steroids suppress your immune system and therefore increase your risk of various infections, which place a demand on your adrenal glands. If your adrenal glands still have some function, you risk sending the signal that they do not need to bother working and you then become dependent on steroids indefinitely. These issues are more pronounced when you are over-medicating and is why you should attempt to find the lowest dose that keeps you healthy.

To adequately treat low cortisol and make the lifestyle changes necessary to improve your body's cortisol output, it is important to understand your body's natural cortisol curve (below). In general, cortisol peaks at 8am, dips at 11 am – 12 pm and again at 2-4 pm, and starts to fall at 8 pm until it nearly zeroes out from midnight – 4 am. Any pharmaceutical treatment should mimic your natural cortisol highs and lows.

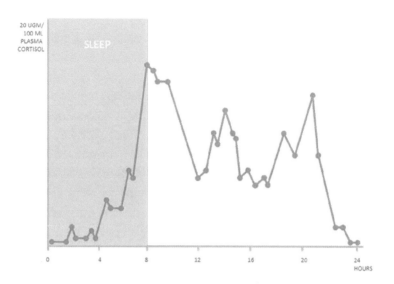

Pharmaceutical Advice

I strongly recommend that you remain highly critical of the variety of pharmaceuticals that will be offered to you and aim to not take any other non-steroid pharmaceuticals. This is because of my experience being prescribed medication that was harmful to my recovery (i.e. beta-blockers that lowered my blood pressure further) and because it is very important that you minimize all side effects that cause your body any stress.

I have read that "hormones at the top of the cascade, such as pregnenolone, have fewer side effects than down-stream hormones such as cortisol. Hormones at the top allow the adrenal to make its own down-stream hormone whereas hormones at the bottom are more potent/ have the greatest potential side effects." While I have also read that this is debatable, I find my cortisol prescription to be very potent...just an extra quarter pill can take me from bed-ridden to gardening.

You should also be critical of the dosing instructions. In my first attempt I was told to only take my prescriptions in the morning because they could cause insomnia close to bedtime. If I am sick near bedtime I do not worry about losing sleep due to extra medication. The outcome is the same – I am going to lose some sleep. This is either because I took medication close to bedtime or because my body is going into crisis without the medication. It has been healthier for me to take some cortisol and lose a little sleep but have a functioning body rather than deprive my body of the cortisol it needs and attempt to sleep through it.

In my second attempt I was told to take my cortisol steroid at ~8 am and ~2 pm. Instead, I have learned to take my prescriptions whenever I need them.

My Story

Stabilization

I was taking 0.5 mg of dexamethasone and 0.1 mg of fludrocortisone daily. However, I would regularly have to take extra steroids as every little stress or ailment was pushing me towards a crisis.

Decent Day	Bad Day
0.75 mg of dexamethasone	1-1.5 mg of dexamethasone
0.1 mg of fludrocortisone	0.1 mg of fludrocortisone

Recovery

After four months I switched to hydrocortisone. After a few weeks of taking 5mg of hydrocortisone and 0.1 mg fludrocortisone at 7:30-8 am and another 2.5 mg of hydrocortisone at 2:30 pm (as instructed), I was still crashing regularly between 10-11 am and having to take another 1.25-2.5 mg.

Decent Day	Bad Day
6.25 mg of hydrocortisone	7.5 mg of hydrocortisone
0.1 mg of fludrocortisone	0.1 mg of fludrocortisone

Recovery/Too Low

During the first month I was taking 2.5 mg of hydrocortisone upon wakening (7:30-8 am) and another 2.5 mg at 11 am to combat the somewhat regular crash symptoms between 10-11 am. After a month on hydrocortisone I began to feel more stable, energetic, and healthy. I was able to reduce my dosage to 2.5 mg of hydrocortisone and 0.05 mg of fludrocortisone upon waking and no second dose for weeks at a time. I also simultaneously increased my life's activities and responsibilities.

Decent Day	Bad Day
2.5 mg of hydrocortisone	5-5.25 mg of hydrocortisone
0.05 mg of fludrocortisone	0.05 mg of fludrocortisone

...Continued

Today

After dropping ~10 lbs. at an alarming rate, noticing that I was losing substantially more hair during shampooing, and admitting that I was fighting a mild daily headache ~2 pm, I confirmed with my endocrinologist that I must be under-dosing. Until I gained back the 10 lbs., I increased my morning dose to 3.75 mg (7:30-8 am) and added an afternoon dose of 1.25 mg at ~2 pm. After gaining back the weight, I brought the morning dose back down to 2.5 mg. I have continued to increase my life's activities and responsibilities.

Decent Day	Bad Day
2.5-3.75 mg of hydrocortisone	5-5.25 mg of hydrocortisone
0.05 mg of fludrocortisone	0.05 mg of fludrocortisone

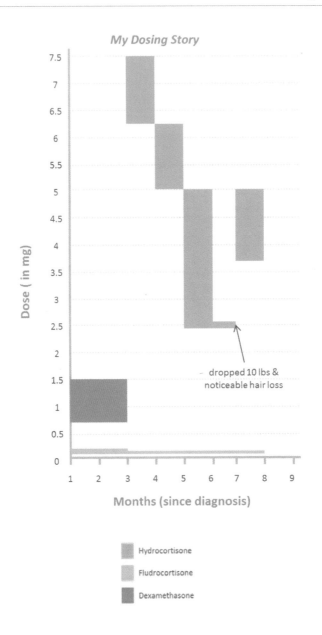

My Dosing Story

Dose (in mg)

Months (since diagnosis)

dropped 10 lbs & noticeable hair loss

Hydrocortisone

Fludrocortisone

Dexamethasone

Commonly Prescribed Steroids

About Dexamethasone

Dexamethasone is simultaneously the best and worst medication you will be on. Dexamethasone is a long-acting corticosteroid that is eliminated by the liver. Importantly, dexamethasone does not interfere with the serum cortisol test you will need and so will probably be your doctor's first treatment choice.

The good news about being long acting is that your body is more reliably getting the signal that you have cortisol available. When you are first being diagnosed and very sick, you will appreciate the stability it provides. The bad news is that it does not mimic your body's normal rising and falling levels of cortisol.

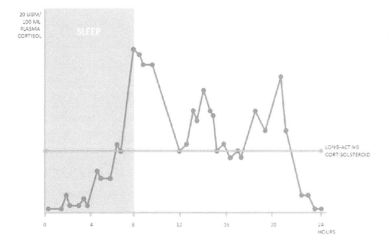

If you're like me, you will start to notice that you do not feel quite "normal" after you have stabilized. Dexamethasone is far more potent than cortisol in its glucocorticoid effect in your body (both in intensity and length) and does not mimic normal production and excretion of cortisol. I noticed that I never had any moments of high energy no matter how I ate or exercised. I felt consistently low-energy throughout the day and was not getting the signal from my body that it was time to fall asleep.

Any synthetic steroid medications that have a similar action to cortisol – such as prednisone, prednisolone, and dexamethasone – may actually cause adrenal insufficiency because their presence in the blood tricks your body into thinking the adrenals can stop producing cortisol. This is why you can never just stop taking steroids – your body will not be trained and ready to make up the difference. It is also important to note that dexamethasone is one of the most common glucocorticoids which cause steroid diabetes.

My Unpleasant Side Effects
Over four months I had a marked increase in facial blemishes and the skin on my forehead and chin was thickening, causing further skin irritation/redness. I kept gaining weight past the weight I had lost during the crises. One month I had the worst PMS I can ever remember, and my periods were different in terms of duration and intensity. In the last month I had a constant yeast infection that required several prescriptions. I suspect I had elevated blood sugar and was also concerned about increasing osteoporosis since I am already in the demographic for it.

About Fludrocortisone

Fludrocortisone replaces aldosterone, which is a mineralocorticoid that influences your salt and potassium balance and therefore blood pressure and fluid balance. Aldosterone tells the kidneys to reabsorb sodium and water and secrete potassium, which results in an increase of blood pressure and blood volume.

While most Addison's patients are prescribed a very low dose, in large doses fludrocortisone inhibits adrenal cortisol secretion, thyroid, and pituitary activity, which is what you are trying to fix in the first place.

I have definitely noticed an improvement in my hydration (I have also been diligent about sports drinks with salt added). I had regular blood draws over several months and noticed my blood went from a pale red color and slow/low volume to scarlet red and a volume that causes the needle hole to actually squirt blood.

My Unpleasant Side Effects
I am not able to attribute any of my side effects to the fludrocortisone.

About Hydrocortisone

Hydrocortisone *is* cortisol. Accordingly, it mimics the body's glucocorticoid effect in both intensity and length. It is more quickly absorbed and secreted than longer-lasting steroids like dexamethasone, meaning you have to take it more than once each day and be disciplined about responding to your body's needs. I switched to hydrocortisone because I hit a plateau after my initial stabilization period. I was still experiencing sick days that were not be remedied by more medication.

I assume that hydrocortisone's more natural signals give the adrenal glands their best chance at recovery and that the shorter half-life means the body could be steroid-free at some point during the day. If it ever becomes possible, I believe this approach will give my adrenals their best chance to function normally. The following graph demonstrates what I believe is happening when I take hydrocortisone at ~8 am and ~11 am. I have no data to back this up and I am sure the amounts are incorrect, but it demonstrates what I feel is happening:

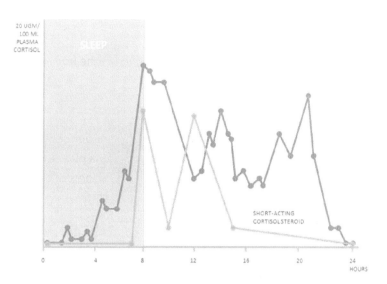

My Unpleasant Side Effects

I immediately developed a skin infection that caused red, swollen bumps around my mouth and nose that lasted for several months and did not respond to naturopathic remedies or the desonide prescription (described below). I also broke out with these bumps each time I increased my hydrocortisone to battle stress.

I am not sure if it is due to the adrenal glands or the steroids, but I caught the first cold that went around work and seemed to have the most severe symptoms. About once a month I suspect a yeast infection and am able to fight it off with naturopathic remedies. Thankfully, I feel "normal" again and have experienced a more normal sleeping pattern. I am getting the signal to go to sleep each night, falling asleep without medication, sleeping more soundly, and feel more refreshed in the morning.

THE BEST THING THAT EVER HAPPENED

The best thing that ever happened to me since my diagnosis was reading the comments in an Addison's blog and discovering that other Addison's patients were setting their alarm ~30 minutes before they would get out of bed to take their steroids. They would take their steroids, go back to bed, and either allow themselves to wake up on their own or get out of bed ~30 minutes later. This conflicted with my prescription's directions, which warned about nausea from taking steroids on an empty stomach.

While I do not agree with alarms for Addison's sufferers, taking my medication when I first wake up naturally and then resting until I feel ready to get out of bed has greatly improved my quality of life. I feel I am starting the day ahead of my symptoms...as though I woke up on my own and have some energy on reserve. When I was waiting to take my medication with breakfast I felt I had to force myself out of bed and that I was starting with an energy deficit. I have never had nausea from this approach, which says a lot for me as mild nausea has been a common theme throughout my life.

Stress Dosing vs. Up Dosing

If you join any support groups you will quickly learn that dosing to respond to events (how much and how often) is a hotly debated topic. Thanks to online forums, I have seen endocrinologists provide wildly different instructions on the topic. For patients taking glucocorticoid hormones on a routine basis, I believe it is necessary to define two very different but equally useful styles of dosing: stress dosing and up dosing.

Stress Dosing

Stress dosing is necessary when experiencing *significant* stress (fever, severe and sudden injury, illness that includes vomiting, diarrhea, or dehydration, etc.). Stress dosing involves taking an extra double to triple dose of the steroid medication to avoid severe consequences. Stress dosing always requires your doctor's input, must be continued until the stress has diminished, and requires tapering off the extra dose. If your symptoms cannot be controlled by stress dosing, go to the nearest medical facility for intravenous steroids and saline.

Up Dosing

Up dosing is necessary when experiencing *mild to moderate* stress (cold without a fever, mild injury, emotional stress, infection, etc.). Up dosing involves taking an extra ¼-½ pill of the steroid medication to avoid mild to moderate consequences. Up dosing can be done without your doctor's input (although you should *always* define your up-dosing strategies with them ahead of time), dosing may or may not be continued until the stress has diminished, and you can return to the normal dose without necessarily needing to taper.

Fortunately and unfortunately, the correct dosing strategy depends on your situation. First and foremost, you need to be acutely aware of your earliest warning signs that you are requiring extra cortisol. It is critical to listen to and respond to your body's needs. What works for one person may not work for you. It is always better to avoid the descent into a crisis by taking an up dose than to descend into a crisis and require a stress dose. Make a plan with your doctor. What amount of steroid can you reasonably take to respond to life's regular stresses? What amount of steroid causes concern and requires your doctor's input?

My Story

I regularly up dose with an extra ¼-½ pill (1.25-2.5 mg) of hydrocortisone to respond to abnormal work stress, emotional stress, head colds, physical overexertion, a very poor night's sleep, or eating something I am sensitive to. I do not taper on or off these small doses; I just take them at will.

After my diagnosis I dropped a mirror on my foot that required three stitches. I consulted the nurse about stress dosing but he was not familiar with Addison's disease and so when he said it was not necessary I ignored his advice. I took another full dose while waiting for my stitches (meaning I had doubled my daily dose – to a total of 7.5 mg) and maintained my double dose for the next 48 hours. I tapered my dose by ¼ pill a day until I was back down to my "normal" daily dose. I am glad I stress dosed – my foot took 3x the recommended healing time even with the extra cortisol.

Additional Steroids

Since hormone treatment is more of an art than a science, you may be prescribed a variety of additional steroids. The steroids below are ones I have had personal experience with, but are by no means "typical" for Addison's treatment or necessary in your particular case. However, just because these hormones are not typical for Addison's treatment does not mean you should not explore them as necessary for your health. Your goal is to achieve homeostasis in all your body's processes so that you are not taxing your adrenal glands.

About DHEA

Dehydroepiandrosterone (DHEA) comes from the adrenal gland and brain and produces male and female sex hormones. DHEA levels begin to decrease after age 30 and more quickly in women.

After a crisis that shouldn't have happened, finding out my estrogen was clinically low, reading that corticosteroids may reduce DHEA levels, and that low DHEA is common in people with hormonal disorders I started taking 25 mg DHEA. From that day on I noticed a more subtle, stable hormonal response. However, after two months of daily DHEA I started to notice some side effects attributable to DHEA and began to cut back my dose. A few weeks later I started seeing an OB/GYN who suspects I may be experiencing estrogen dominance and I decided to stop the DHEA altogether.

My Unpleasant Side Effects
After two months without side effects I began to notice itchy scalp, smaller breasts, and acne (important to note this facial blemish was different than the dermatitis described below).

About Progesterone
Progesterone is a primary precursor in the biosynthesis of the adrenal corticosteroids. Without adequate progesterone, synthesis of the cortisones is impaired and the body turns to alternate pathways. Steroid progesterone is very similar to the hormone progesterone that is produced by the ovaries.

Progesterone does not need to be taken every day; usually on days 15-26 of each menstrual cycle. After testing low for progesterone in a blood test and seeing an OB/GYN who suspects I may be experiencing estrogen dominance, I began taking 100 mg of progesterone daily.

My Unpleasant Side Effects
After a few days I realized it was making me markedly drowsy and began taking it at night. It did improve my ability to sleep deeply, but after one week I experienced very unusual cramping and vaginal bleeding and stopped taking it. I also suspect it caused a sore throat, neck, and back muscles. It is important to note that progesterone increases your risk of cardiovascular disorders and breast and uterine cancer. I continued to spot for nearly two weeks, then did not experience spotting for ~3 days, then spotted again for ~5 days.

About Birth Control

After the negative experience with just progesterone I was more convinced that I should trust my test results that show I was low in both estrogen and progesterone. I found that identified with more symptoms of low estrogen than high estrogen. I began Lutera Tablets 28's (a.k.a. birth control). These contain Ethinyl estradiol (a derivative of E2) and levonorgestrel (synthetic progesterone).

It is important to note that birth control pills can increase your blood cortisol level, but I am not able to say what this means for the Addison's patient as the long-term effects are not known. Oestrogen increases non-protein-bound, protein-bound, and total plasma cortisol levels. These increases are dependent on the dose of oestrogen and are not usually seen with progesterone-only or `low-dose' oestrogen birth control.

My Unpleasant Side Effects

I had a runny nose that caused a mild sore throat for the first ~3 days. I also developed a painful case of perioral dermatitis (a.k.a. steroid induced rosacea) that required antibiotics to clear up.

About Desonide Cream

I was prescribed desonide topical 0.05% – a steroid – to combat the red, swollen bumps that developed around my mouth and nose. While not likely an issue, it is known that applying a topical steroid to a large surface area (>30%) can cause hypothalamic-pituitary-adrenal axis suppression.

My Unpleasant Side Effects
The cream added to the oiliness of my skin. After two months, it never completely cleared up my dermatitis. It seems to only be effective if used sparingly, and even then it does not completely remedy the blemishes.

My Story

My most stubborn side effect to date has been perioral dermatitis (a.k.a. steroid-induced rosacea). It started when I switched to hydrocortisone and I unsuccessfully managed it for three months before it became painful to open my mouth.

I tried supplementing my immune system, Abreva (10% docosanol), Desitin (40% zinc oxide), Aveeno (1% hydrocortisone), Polysporin (500 units bacitracin/10,000 units polymyxin B), anti-fungal liquid (25% undecylenic acid), and then prescription 0.05% Desonide lotion, 5% acyclovir ointment, and 1% Metronidazole.

Completely changing my skin maintenance habits and the 1% Metronidazole showed some promise, but I did not heal until I took a several week course of antibiotics (tetracycline). I consider myself healed, except for some daily redness immediately after taking my steroids.

I do not let anything unnatural touch my face (no sodium lauryl sulfate, fluoride, or other ingredients I cannot pronounce), I use a separate towel just for my face, tone with apple cider vinegar or witch hazel, and use coconut oil as a moisturizer. I use the 1% Metronidazole for maintenance.

Naturopathic Treatments

For any ailment, a holistic approach to your health can prevent conditions that worsen your symptoms. As always, a diet and level of exercise that is healthy for you will ward off many of the culprits that contribute to adrenal fatigue. Your naturopathic remedies should aim to reduce inflammation, relieve stress, support your immune system, and relieve side effects from your other medication. *However, it is important to understand that even bio-available, otherwise-nourishing supplements can stimulate your adrenal glands.*

The sheer amount of naturopathic remedies available for adrenal fatigue is overwhelming and the data behind the recommendations varies significantly. Further, multi-ingredient supplements can contain ingredients that counter-act other supplements you are taking. I wrote this section in the hopes that it represents those naturopathic remedies that are best supported by studies and are least likely to have adverse effects.

- Probiotics
    - Healthy digestive tracts filter out harmful bacteria, toxins, chemicals, and other waste products and take in nutrients from food and water. Maintaining a proper balance in your digestive tract benefits your entire body, but most importantly it supports the proper functioning of your immune system.
    - *Take a probiotic with each steroid dose to avoid nausea and increase uptake of the steroid.*

- B12 shots
  - Vitamin B deficiencies – and most importantly a B12 deficiency – are common with adrenal gland issues. B12 is important for normal functioning of the brain, nervous system, formation of blood, and is involved in the metabolism of every cell of the human body. B12 deficiency symptoms can mimic Addison's, including as weakness, fatigue, light-headedness, rapid heartbeat and breathing, and pale skin. It may also cause easy bruising or bleeding, stomach upset, weight loss, and diarrhea or constipation.
  - *B12 should be administered by injection as patients with poor functioning bodies cannot absorb vitamin B12 taken by mouth.*
- AdrenaCort
  - There are many options for adrenal gland extracts from slaughtered animals. These adrenal glands contain adrenal hormones (the amount of which varies from batch to batch and animal to animal) that, when ingested, are recognized by your body and treated like your own hormones.

    Like all herbal supplements, there seems to be a lack of definitive research about AdrenaCort's effectiveness. However, even if do not buy into the idea of eating another animal's adrenal hormones, AdrenaCort does contain vitamins and minerals shown to support adrenal function and boost hormone production and energy levels – magnesium, zinc, vitamin B, licorice and vitamin C.

Magnesium, for example, is often deficient under stress, is essential for nearly all energy-producing activities, and helps your body take up other important nutrients like 5-HTP, but unfortunately also reduces your sodium levels and blood pressure.

o *Start all supplements on the lowest dose and increase only after you're certain you aren't experiencing any negative side effects.*

My Story

I have had success with the supplement AdrenaCort, but suspect it was over-stimulating my adrenal glands in the recommended dosage. AdrenaCort contains vitamin B5, which is known to stimulate adrenal hormones.

After an Addisonian crisis that should not have happened (I knew my diagnosis, had been successfully managing my symptoms for several months, and had already doubled my prescription medication in an attempt to avoid the crisis), I reduced the amount I was taking by half. I am sure my other lifestyle changes have contributed to the outcome, but I have not had a crisis since reducing my supplement intake.

I regularly take a second look at all I am ingesting (keeping a journal is crucial to remembering all those details you need to make informed decisions). This review often causes me to reduce or change my supplement and prescription routines.

- Hawthorn extract
    - Hawthorn extract reduces blood vessel tension (supporting your ability to regulate blood pressure and fluid balance); increases oxygen in the blood; relieves heart palpitations and chest tightness by decreasing the resistance of blood circulation; atherosclerosis; reduces the formation of plaque in the blood vessels, reduces LDL ("poor") cholesterol; is an antioxidant; and boosts restful sleep (tea form is best).
    - *Hawthorn can lower your blood pressure. If you are experiencing noticeably low blood pressure you may want to skip a dose and increase your Himalayan pink salt intake.*
- 5-HTP
    - 5-HTP helps you manage stress by raising serotonin levels in the brain, which regulates mood and anxiety, improves sleep, appetite, and pain sensation.
    - *Take 5-HTP at night as you do not need anything adding to the fatigue you already feel all day.*
- Licorice root extract
    - In order of importance to adrenal fatigue, licorice:
        - Inhibits the enzyme that inactivates cortisol and allows cortisol access to the mineralcortoid receptors, triggering an increased retention of sodium and a lowering of potassium

- - Boosts immune system chemicals, contains antioxidants, and stops the growth of many bacteria
  - Contains phytoestrogens that can perform some of the functions of the body's natural estrogens
  - Lowers stomach acid levels and relieves irritation, inflammation, and spasm in the digestive tract
  - Is anti-allergenic effect, possibly through its ability to improve resistance to stress
  - Reduces irritation and inflammation in the respiratory system
  - Increases bile flow in the liver
  - Lowers cholesterol levels
  - *Licorice root can increase blood pressure so do not take it if you have high blood pressure/are experiencing an episode of high blood pressure.*

- Lysine
  - Lysine has been proven to reduce stress/anxiety, increase intestinal absorption of calcium (which combats osteoporosis caused by steroid use), increase muscle mass, and lower glucose (to help with hyperglycemia you may have from steroid use).

  - *Lysine can also lower cortisol levels in the blood, which is good for the decent into adrenal fatigue (when cortisol is over-produced) but may not be beneficial for full-blown adrenal fatigue (when you are cortisol-deficient).*

- Zinc

    o Zinc supports the proper functioning of the immune and digestive systems, control of blood sugar levels, reduction of stress, energy, and an increased rate of healing for acne and wounds. Zinc is often deficient under stress.

    o *Zinc can stimulate the adrenal glands and should be taken conservatively to ensure the adrenal glands are resting.*

Doctor Advice

See two doctors simultaneously – an endocrinologist and a naturopathic doctor. Your endocrinologist will ensure your organs are protected and your naturopath is going to ensure your whole person is thriving. My endocrinologist looked at my adrenal glands in detail – structure, function, and signals coming to and from it. My naturopath assessed the entire picture – food sensitivities, micronutrient deficiencies, sleep patterns, and other things that may be keeping my whole self from thriving. My endocrinologist quickly identified the Addison's and then my naturopath identified a B12 deficiency, very low estrogen, potential diet deficiencies, and potentially harmful lifestyle habits.

To know if you have the right doctor, ask them what they think about adrenal fatigue. Is it real or a hoax? If they summarily dismiss it as a hoax, ask them why and consider a new doctor. Even if you do not believe in adrenal fatigue, you deserve a fully attentive physician that will investigate all possible adrenal issues, not just the well-documented ones. Is your doctor willing to take phone calls and emails with questions about seemingly minute details? This is a disease that is different for each person. Are they willing to meet your personal needs?

You will be repeatedly accused of being depressed or suffering from anxiety. Unfortunately a symptom of Addison's is generalized anxiety and depression and the easy answer is a mental disorder. Remain confident that you're at the doctor because your body – not your mind – is trying to tell you something.

Crises

Remember that your adrenal glands are not able to help you recover and you must manage your recovery with your prescriptions. Your best management strategy is to become overly familiar with your earliest warning symptoms.

At first I was only aware of my more severe symptoms that presented themselves when I was close to a crisis (see sidebar). As I became more familiar with my condition I started recognizing the much more subtle, earlier symptoms that would indicate I was heading for a crisis.

Instead of reacting to more severe symptoms later, I react to the earliest symptoms I can identify and take some extra prescription medication. Within the limits of your prescribed medication range, I have found it never hurts to take more medication (0.25 mg at a time) to avoid either the crisis symptoms, or the stress of wondering if you are experiencing crisis symptoms.

My Story

My trajectory to a crisis generally follows this symptom pattern:

Racing heart

Sweating/sweaty palms

Fatigue

Burning/dry eyes

Nausea

Uncomfortable bowel movement

Inability to concentrate

Dehydration

Muscle weakness

Cold extremities

Labored breathing

Abdominal pain

Slurred speech

Pre-syncope

What to Tell Your Friends & Family

"My adrenal glands don't work properly, which means I don't properly respond to or recover from physical or emotional stress. I have to take steroids to replace the hormones my adrenal glands no longer supply. Hormone management is more of an art than a science, and until I figure out my personal health management plan I will at times be fatigued, irritable, nauseous, and have trouble thinking clearly. I need your help slowing down my life and allowing myself to be in full recovery mode. If there is an emergency where I'm unconscious, please let the medical staff know my adrenal glands don't work and I need steroids immediately."

Medical Alert Bracelet

Based on what I've read, the most recognizable text you should get on your medical bracelet is "Adrenal insufficiency; steroid reliant." However, remember that this is not a common and recognizable disorder, so you'll want to make sure your friends and family are informed in case of an emergency.

Made in the USA
Lexington, KY
07 March 2015